Covodes

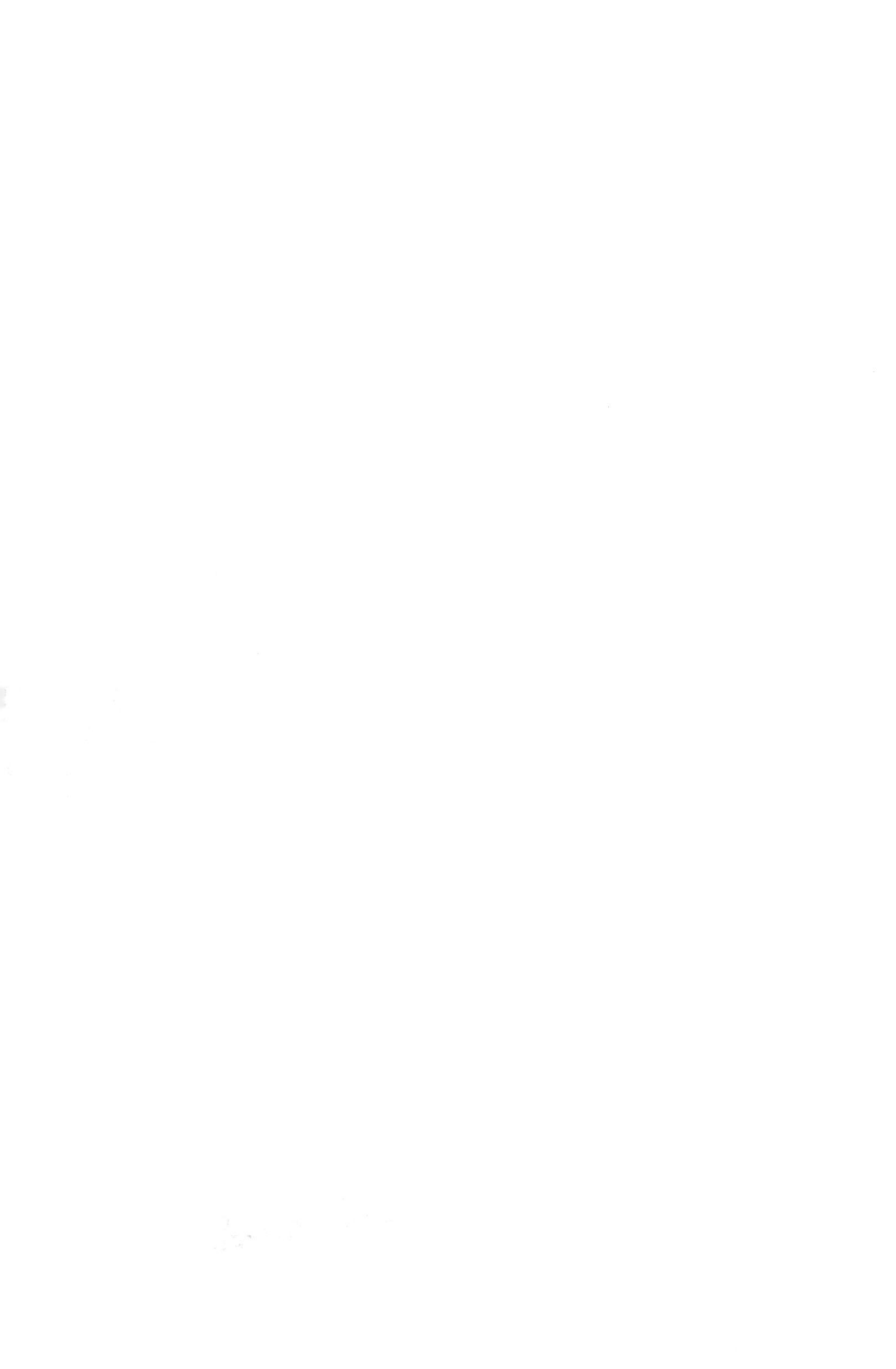

Covodes

Poems

by

Robert Hampson

Artery Editions 2021

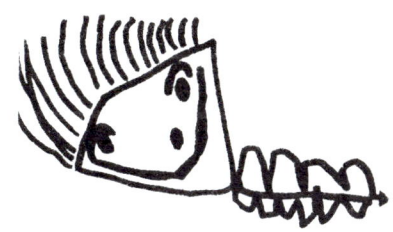

Published by:

Artery Editions
Our Lady's House
43 Carisbrooke Road
St Leonard's-on-Sea
East Sussex
UK, TN38 0JT

Artery Express
ISBN/EAN: 1871671078/9781871671070

Art Edition,
Signed, 20 copies, Poems by Robert Hampson, Music by Joanna Levi
and Art by John Vernon Lord

ISBN/EAN: 1871671086/9781871671087

British Library Cataloguing-in-Publication Data.
A catalogue record for this book is available from the British Library

Dedication

to

Gerlinde Roder-Bolton, my companion in Lockdown

Editor: Patricia Hope Scanlan

Graphic Design & Typeset by Clare Davey
Printed by Fastprinting, St Leonard's-on-Sea.
Cover Design *Untitled* © Robert Hampson, 2021

An Edition of 250 copies with CD Recording of *Covodes* read by Robert Hampson, Cello Music, titled *Suite 1 for Solo Cello*, composed and performed by Joanna Levi. Recording and sound design by Cameron Macgregor

A signed numbered Art Edition of 20 copies of *Covodes* by Robert Hampson, with tipped in art works by John Vernon Lord. Included are the CD recordings of *Covodes*, *Suite 1 for Solo Cello* by Joanna Levi.

Bandcamp Version:

A Digital Version of the *Covodes* Recording can be purchased (for £5.00) via arteryeditions.bandcamp.com
All rights reserved.

Acknowledgements:

Some of these poems have appeared in *Rewilding: An Ecopoetic Anthology* (Crested Tit Collective, 2020); *Covid & Poetry*, edited by Anthony Calescu; *Molly Bloom*, edited by Aidan Semmens; Lyndon Davies and his magazine *Junctionbox*. I am grateful to these editors for showing earlier versions of these poems. I am also grateful to *The Guardian* and *The Observer* for the articles and reports which, over the last year, have gone into this mix. Articles by Sarah Perry and Laura Cummings have a particular role in the sequence.

Thanks:

Artery Editions would like to thank all those who have assisted in getting *Covodes* together for publication. A special thanks to Christopher Beckett, Libby Musso Dacre, Gabriel Wishart, John Vernon Lord, Cameron Macgregor and Clare Davey. Thanks too to Jeremy Reed, Hope Wishart, Peter Ellson, Benedict Wishart, Paul Khimasia Morgan, Barnaby Wyther, Holly Saunders and Sophie Sparkes.

Previous Artery Editions Publications:

Spiral (2004) Poems by Fanny Howe, Music by Ken Edwards, Art by Tom Raworth, Compiled by Patricia Hope Scanlan, CD with Live Recording

Gifts received (2007) Poem by Lee Harwood, Music by Birdie Hall, Art by Francis Wishart. CD: Reading by Lee Harwood, Soundscape by Birdie Hall

Κοπσστια – *Heartloss-Cuts* (2008) Poems by Nikos Stangos, Art by Jasper Johns & Patricia Hope Scanlan. (A3 Perspex Art Book, A2 Perspex Art Book, Art Book)

Oh, Lac... Oh, Lake... (2008) Poems by Pierre Martory, Translations by John Ashbery, Art by Francis Wishart, Edited by Eugene Richie and Olivier Brossard, Compiled by Patricia Hope Scanlan

Scheme (2021) dedicated to Panna Grady O'Connor. Poems by Philip O'Connor, Essay John Berger, Film (BFI), *Captain Busby The Even Tenour of Her Ways* (Director Ann Wolff, 1967), Art by Andrzej Maria Borkowski, edited by Patricia Hope Scanlan

Uplift: A Samizdat for Lee Harwood (2008) by his friends Tribute Edition, with Music Composition from Birdie Hall, Edited by Patricia Hope Scanlan, Assistant Editor Tim Weston

Strictly Illegal Poems (2011) by John Wieners, Art by Gilbert & George, Selected & Introduced by Jeremy Reed, Biography by George F. Butterick, Edited by Patricia Hope Scanlan, General and A2 Art Edition

Thinking of Li Po (1995) Poems by Philip O'Connor, Art by Aneela Majid & illustration by Monika Duda, ISBN 978 1 871671 11 7 Artery Editions/Ink Sculptors/Cult Productions

Forthcoming Artery Editions include:

Le Madame Poems and Recordings by Deborah Levy, Mine Kaylan, Patricia Hope Scanlan & Art by Louise Bourgeois, Introduced by Griselda Pollock. Recordings & Soundscapes by Joseph Young, Introduced by Paul Khimasia Morgan

Brighton Blues A Poetry Tribute to the Poet Lee Harwood by Jeremy Reed, Art by Derek Jarman, Recording of Lee Harwood's *Landscapes* by Stream Records. *Brighton Blues* also features an Essay by Lee Harwood on the Poet F.T. Prince & Letters from Lee Harwood to Jeremy Reed, & from John Ashbery to Lee Harwood, & Poems from Anne Waldman, & Patricia Hope Scanlan. Film Tribute from Patricia Hope Scanlan, *Starlings over Hastings Pier*, 2021

Pente Poems by John Wieners, Art by William Blake & John Cage, edited & compiled by Patricia Hope Scanlan

Reprint *Oh, Lac... Oh, Lake...* (2008) Poems by Pierre Martory, Translations by John Ashbery, Art by Francis Wishart, Edited by Eugene Richie and Olivier Brossard, Compiled by Patricia Hope Scanlan

A Hole in the Sky Tribute to Gustav Metzger and Yoko Ono, Work DVD by Patricia Hope Scanlan

Explosive Cornelia Parker, Interview with Patricia Hope Scanlan, Work DVD

Contents

nevermind

so, what's the damage?

here there's just dust

& grime

& cobwebs

stretch from the doorframe

to the ground

we could have set up a meet

with the friends of Kurt Cobain

Covode 1: the people's disease

I.

It's the bright sunny start of april

& the delegates assess the outbreak

there was no procedure the statistics

are only the iceberg's tip the swab

samples less than fascinating

the professor cruises the silent university

this is a narrative of entry

into an unwilling host kismet

written into the antibody response

II.

never take your companions for granted

notice the stress points in the culture industry

the patterns it takes during lock-down

expose the limits of live performance

empty supermarket shelves &

packed-full basement freezers

its another nail-biter for retailers

as the online grocery drama determines

where the supply line hasn't been able to cope

III.

24-hour stores with their wage-slave

distribution models & click-bait services

the online logjam limits online shoppers

so many slots so many stained pages per order

the pressure on hospitals the closure of schools

the shredding of ministerial reputations

at an alarming rate at a warming rate

IV.

I was an accredited researcher

      ready at any time

           to deliver serosurveys

I was an experienced serosurveiller

      a veteran of the housing estates

           & the outlying suburbs

the violence of the policy-makers

lingers in the blood long after recovery

V.

our chances mutated four seasons ago

the dismantling of public health systems

to let the virus rip through the populace

through care-homes & factories

low-paid workers compelled to use public transport

Covode 2: a planetary testimony

I.

eventually it will all even out

sure you can't actually feel

a whole lot happier beforehand

incomplete information doesn't help

but now we are all like brothers

it's 3.a.m. in Berlin

& the band strikes up 'Big City Nights'

II.   indifference

this is the second life

this is a social media PR task

Martian clouds & dust-storms

& no magnetic field to protect us from radiation

this is the year of the singing winds

much has remained hot & gorgeous

like edicts by tweet from a reptile brain

we were not re-assured by the first close-up

it revealed a dead world – no trace of joy

just a robot rover called Indifference

it's hard to be sure, maybe we ARE all Martians

III.   **curiosity**

the robot detects (tweet) a degradation

of the infrastructure how we phrase sentences

as victims or victors for observers in Beijing

there's poverty on Mars & lavish

handclapping as heroes die

without the right equipment (tweet)

perhaps life does mean wearing bin-bags?

we lie awake worrying

only to be sold the same steroid regime

huddled over in my Brexit t-shirt

studying the uncertain map of the planet

as a private-equity acquisition

IV.   emotional well-being

just hop into the next crafted confection

cold war history matters, nuclear arsenals,

rip-tides of mental confusion from duff intelligence

'well-being trumps love' says Beavers

eagles & pine-martens return as rewilding

the new autobiography of the species

she has her own butterfly, he is the

white stork re-introduced into West Sussex

she loves elk – so marriages go

like other numbers games

V.   **perseverance**

no matter, if you keep thinking correctly

these are the seeds of resistance

be prepared for direction (for decades to come)

& no way of leaving or making peace

the fetch rover will collect soil samples

this may be its greatest gift

how can I craft a table?

how did I make such a great deal

go wrong?

we should have vetoed it, the writing

already on the wall, coronavirus exercising

this mid-march marriage

in mid-stride after he dug his heels in

one talks about the need to sit on the fence

the next is calling reject

VI. ingenuity

if you are a model husband, so much the better

she had had a political upbringing

he wasn't one to show charm & fun

slipped more quickly than a metal bed-frame

on a tiled floor

seas & lakes have been turned on

for the start-up he joined on Mars

who would want a freelance-writer's income?

the robot has been diagnosed with bizarre bristles

no-one knows what it is

the Head of the Atmospheric Services thinks

nothing is quite so cynical

as a flypast during lockdown

VII.   a picture of two lives (by Anthony Fauci)

he's speaking for the right & he's not

hostile to science on his previous planet

all the core was molten & disinfectant

could be injected like a magnetic field

to protect against radiation

however life evolves, it all happens

after the fact & the Department probes

to close down knowledge of what it did

on return to Earth, everything that is

proves to be the case, no-one knows

what to do next, it's usually a chance

to find life on Mars, to land a craft,

zap rocks with an ultra-violet laser,

to find lost Americans – or save the president

if you have money, the photographer said,

who wants to see you party as a ghost?

Covode 3: the little lockdown: a synthetic meditation

4 pina bausch & the chicks

I.

we measure the event in terms of droplets

we develop an app.   place

ambiguous lumps of flesh on the table

we begin to understand the microwave oven

though these things are elusive

we watch them come back to life

II.

coughing all night /   & panting

waiting for the barrage / & the flare of gas

world wars make / poor comparators

when the minister /   misuses the statistics

we embrace all that this entails

III.

a midnight dance through the castle gardens

a choir with polar bears on an ice-floe

a best-selling paperback of the pandemic

an earth fit for filming

(set sometime in the past)

IV.

the cruise ship left in 1995, bound for the former Confederate states, Hawaii & Polynesia with guest-lecturers along for the ride. to begin with everything went to plan: slides were shown, questionnaires handed out, CDs were burned

V.

heavy logging in the Amazon

immense fires in Siberia

& a virus in the editing suite

a maverick geographer

offers independent help & advice

It's a nice standard star

with a self-regulating system

it's an engineer's dream of music

new species flourish

all we are is a food supply

VI.

I can think of a lot worse workplaces. we had 3 good meals per day, a woman at night, & sunbathing on the back-deck.

a lone dancer in a darkened room. 350 forms of exhaustion in the way of entertainment.

VII.

tracing contacts is like going back to high school

I felt we were being institutionalised

trying to work out which way to go

one of them says something

along the lines of: is this covid-19?

next stop: Tahiti

we tried to negotiate with ports for access

we were dubbed traitors

we even got banned from the radio

our future was stolen from us

VIII.

it was a story about a town council

they consulted walked around

built new housing on brown-field sites

the entire affair was designed

to contain social unrest

the terrible harvest of a generation

it was the story of a local girl

doomed to dance until she dropped

it was a story of insistent daubings

& herbal highs

they did not know they were susceptible

it was the smell of the plague

it was the kicking-off point

                            for art & music

IX.

all we needed / was a bit of money

to develop a detector

all we wanted / was to fill the gaps

to break the line / of transmission

all we wanted / was a precise measure

X.

some got to play bingo & see shows. when they learned the
medication was running out, they made their own creative
choices: stoic, angry, sorrowful. the stars followed suit & became
more intense

they said: we're just one big happy family really

she invited them to perform. she wanted them to be Dutch,
Germans, Americans. we said: this could be a handful

used & abused by everybody, we were good to go. No-one
on board got locked into their cabins. she kept us up-to-date
through video-conferencing.

Covode 4: the pleasure dome

4 dido harding

'remember me & don't forget my name'

I.   experiments in architecture

this structure exists / only to protect the richest

a closed system for the apocalypse

with lounge chairs & picnic tables

II.   level 2: operational domain

space means a huge white leather sofa

it's daytime & the screens change automatically

this is a submarine kept on high alert

we take the lift up to the upper-deck

III. geo-protection

the residents need all this stuff

luxury is the key to survival

along with regular spraying

& varying degrees of fumigation

everyone needs to work, generally

that's just human nature

fear has demoralised us

the sun on my face & the smell of burning

when countries descend into a haze of smoke

the question arises whether the money

might have been better spent

the three of us ended up in Argentina

IV. infection rates

can you imagine a low-contact lunch-time

follow the food & the medication

trade routes & supply chains

susceptible to disruption

V.   flashpoints

we walk into a bedroom

with a flat-screen tv

& the screen goes black

a balcony with a railing

& sliding glass doors

nuclear warheads provide

the life-support system

ready for use above

or below the surface

VI.   surround sound

despite the deaths, low-key depression

& incipient cabin-fever

she comes over every day

to check the mail

there was no chance of fixing

the world that we broke

we could only hope

to bamboozle & deceive

while we build

these underground redoubts

social networks are fucked

we live in a real

hermetically-sealed environment

with streaming of trees & grass

on all the screens

I returned with my seafood

this isn't about infected people

people get bored / & break things

this is about covert trade deals

the survival of / an economic system

while wild fires spread / across the pacific

VII.   **what comes next**

we must remember the code

for submarine-launched missiles

we have gas-masks, first-aid kits, pepper-sprays

thermal, night & full-spectrum weapons

this is safe, self-contained, comprehensive

this is a project in communal isolation

designed to survive a nuclear winter

we have learned a lot about triggers

you can imagine food disappearing

but not weaponry

poor oxygen levels have led to

disappointing crop yields

a resurgence of right-wing populism

& territorial rivalries

we go back to the lift

& hit the amnesia button

VIII.   buying into the bunker

nuclear-powered nations / can advertise their missiles

& fertilise the soil / for deeper arsenals

in future, words will have no value

we will have the potential to revive

the things we care about

a great library of sound recordings

& the ubiquitous forms / of authoritarian power

IX.   before disquiet, disinformation

I have had the same feeling before

in different compartments bars

& hotels with high-end appliances

it is dark outside

we were duped with a test & trace system

that doesn't work

that abandons the poorest communities

my job is to help

come on

I'll show you restrictions

X.   test-fire: moral duty

there is a bar on miracle cures

honey, garlic, hydroxychloroquine

on governments spreading their lies

everyone's baking bread & taking yoga classes

everyone's studying online during lockdown

we've had a taste of things to come

we need to get used to this new routine

the latest round of provocations

this could be a mistake

a high-tec high-risk arms race

this could end very badly

I remember the first satellite in orbit

that sense of wonder has subsided

Covode 5: double exposure

I.

we have bleached all the surfaces

in the apartment

it's what we used to call

documentation

self-portraits on the way to school

taking shifts / in a makeshift bed

cowboy hats in Berlin bars

now hygiene rules

& we wash our hands / in medical alcohol

II.

we cut up magazines / to confront the virus

we swap our accessible life

for a cheap & creative / melancholia

III.

his collaborators are all suits

lockdown celebrities

their words come out slurred

we try not to read / the opinion pieces

there's a spectre / in the transmission

it's unnerving to think /this could be the end

IV.

she came back home

from lockdown at the factory

hot & sweaty

in the new merchandise

hair shaved close to the scalp

V.

we hadn't been out for days

we were banned from Instagram

for inciting panic

we removed our masks / to talk on the phone

there were tears in the fabric

& the music suddenly went quiet

we live by the thermometer

& go to bed in the afternoons

Covode 6: risky business

4 sarah perry

I.   last week, to begin with

we thought it

was curtains

the gates were

locked & the

fatality rate

cast a shadow

on hand-rails

& coffee-cups

II.   climactic calamity

I'd entered the new headquarters

she laughed when I explained

all I'd ever wanted

was written into that contract

the result was negative

to play so fast & so hard

to question authority

the name change wrote itself

III.   civic unrest

we should wash our hands

of economic meltdown

& a collapsing ecosystem

we should concentrate

on clothing sales

or the last of the Kardashians

IV.   when the children were immune

the risk was a short-term lock-in

& the loss of 'loved ones'

(no-one mentions the unloved)

we stay inside

the structures of racism

where all men flash binary

for the sake of the chancellor

V.   behind the scenes

I can't dictate these / artistic departures

the espresso machine / has nothing to apologise for

we have a research facility / to study regret

among the super-rich

I can't suppress / that background guitar

Kansas is a supermarket

& the company psychologist

has nothing to apologise for either

VI. a wilful dereliction

she does not talk to the sisters

of the intangibles of love

these are the calculable risks

the odds of injury

the death of a marriage

VII. shouldn't we be doing something?

it's all traced back

to the almost imperceptible

dust over the windows

the usual diplomatic

war of words

is a constant risk

a car journey might involve

incalculable consequences

business can be quantified

but what about friendship

& having fun?

Covode 7: a stranger cluster

I.

nobody wanted to own yesterday

now everybody wants to own tomorrow

we'd been watching old movies

mainly online

she'd had a video-conference

some investigative reporter

out of shot, my concentration

started spinning its wheels

II.

we got the report   mother died yesterday

or maybe the day before

so I was doing this court-case in Louisville

it was the start of another angry week

& I was doing some of that /Kentucky attorney jive

don't look at me like that

III.

I had a dream, a recurring dream

a prime dream

we could cultivate customers abroad

a new golden age in South-east Asia

only this time I would take the lead

in a tactical & purely spiritual sense

IV.

this was the face that launched

a thousand satellites

faint flashing objects

in the field of view

V.

the conference market / had adopted his platform

how proud she is of him

the entire cast of *Friends*

                              carried him to the meeting

VI.

he had texted / till his eyes glazed over

we had to rescue all the old lines from irrelevance
after swearing allegiance to the company

a whole bunch of users
linked courtesy of laptops

VII.

he was born into topics like toxic
waste & systemic white privilege

potential brutalism taken up as a child
with other inherited investments

he had the power / to make connections

now the captains can speak / ship to ship

VIII.

a party invitation, our own unaided invite

sent out by zoom

a human-world get-together

though it's mostly customers

no-one remembers the relative

smoothness of those satellites

as they floated into the night sky

soon there will be no China

& not a single state university

in the whole sad country

Covode 8: the liberation of Paris

i.m.
juliette greco

I.

across town at the Gaslighter

it's the last night of a 17-year marriage

we could not convey the original

for the standard *chanson* audience

we had tried to avoid the punk apocalypse

the erosion of the event horizon

II.

her mother returned to work

she vowed never to forgive

those who had investigated her

it's an open wound

inside all of us

locked in this war of attrition

we have the responsibility

never to forgive them

& never to forget

III.

the right to live

the right to work safely

the right to think, to laugh

to love whomsoever we want

the right to statutory sick leave

IV.

senior officials turned up tonight

as customers

with a taste for the West Midlands

& plans to return staff to work

V.

these measures would be just that second world wide white shirt
& tie cock a hoop & her with her long dark hair & black digital files
communicating with her soulful eyes streaming data as is the way
with *chanteuses* playing someone's tin-eared sounds some of the
take-down repertoire for office-based employment against these
small turns of phrase & their associated musicality a gravitas born
at the Hotel Pont Royale

VI.

they can test & trace work flow from the off, show more data to
the head manager

the guttural noise that means the crowing that staff will continue
to work

the office is full of stuff highly regulated and socially distanced

VII.

some companies may lack warmth

their employees let you hear

their concern about former benefits

the government's priorities will not change

scanning official figures for the working population

monitoring a month of lockdown tweets

reading between the lines

for ethnic background & class

Covode 9: synchronicities

I.   flatlining

the americans agreed

it was working well

we declined to comment

it was justified

II.   pitch-dark

red lights flash on the console

there's trouble with our tiny capsule

there's always a procedure

& when nothing else works

there is always the screwdriver

III.   dropping like flies

I write this in some confusion

he has not learned his lesson

he has no idea / what is happening

IV.   final approach

and it had all been going so well

a double thumbs-up from Kazakhstan

then he peeled his mask off

before locking onto the dock

*there's danger & I'm creeping softly forwards, I don't know, 20 metres
away, close enough, to damage your lives, the space station's cluttered,
our orbit has just begun*

V.   forlorn & stranded

to take the trouble

with a screwdriver

or a bolt-cutter

to break open

the ship's lockers

the consequences are

enormous

to prevent an outbreak

to send a message

to my former self

students of neurology

describe this as

cognitive teaching

to get some shopping

& watch tv

becomes a challenge

to the point that

the impulse was

essentially human

VI. POTUS

Trump was giving trouble

both sides admitted that

they are like ships

embedded in ice

or major cities

with something to hide

Trump was going

experimental

antiviral drugs

& dexamethadone

another surprise

was the armoured car

Trump was in crisis

on the bridge of the White House

& not about to step down

VII.   location data

while some have socially distanced

& some have security flaws

among a wave of cognitive symptoms

forgotten addresses names unknown

'vulnerable' is not a medical term

we recognise

VIII.   feeling good

the disrupters who revel

on oxygen & outrage

require another diagnosis

we don't know if it's a problem

or just the steroids

survivors from the think tank

fear meltdown

meanwhile he says he's perfect

IX.   a sensitive area

we have listed the symptoms

from the website

migraine numbness

birthdays

smart sex-toys

that can be operated remotely

& potentially hacked

X.   the end of the commune

it was going so well

until the white coats

went ballistic

they loom large

in pathology

they carry us over

the back of

synchronicity

the signs flash on

it quickly becomes

all about him

his own political

reality show

Covode 10: bang to eternity

I.

the sound of a sceptical / espresso machine

it's the same aggressive course

a blitzkrieg of tweets

that shocked even these / northern watchers

as boutique narcissism / killed more than the virus

II.

there's local lockdowns / but that's ok

as long as MPs & advisers / stick to the rules

local lockdowns / could not have been avoided

don't get lost in the science / get out there

as far as we know / there's no bottom line

III.

in reality, the same information

but the day is redefined

an indefinite future

though time is running out

in visions of final evaporation

IV.

we can imagine a universe

in which Trump has vanished

the immensity of this

potential universe

is none other than

the inauguration

of the infinite future

V.

he couldn't just / break his own rules

on isolation

looking at them *en masse*

it was possible to see

what thousands had already seen

concentric rings in the sky

& the end of another

conspiracy theory

VI.

the university is dark

there are no customers today

& there will be none

there will be no more universities

just silence

we have gone through

the photographs in his portfolio

his idea is to adopt a dog

or perhaps a tiger

VII.

the staff are now in discussions with that tinpot Mussolini, with
sharp tweets & retweets, not strictly negotiating, but sturdy
anglo-saxon expletives, that breath-taking division between
'somewheres', testing positive, breaking the rules of intimacy with
things & discontents, & no sign of anything for 'anywheres'

VIII.

clusters of galaxies recede at increasing speeds, stars are extinguished, everything reduced to a few black holes, & then the singularity recurs

someone called Einstein the C- word, angry working-class words

we end up evaporating, nothing left, but a trace of light for all eternity

Covode 11: an eco-system south of Portland

(recorded live)

4 bruce springsteen

4 walt whitman

I.   a warning

we were having a word

when out of nowhere

leaves swirled around us

the tormented air

turned blue to dirty grey

we shut down

our networked world

the new moon

had disappeared

the algorithm was

suddenly tangible

we held tight

II.   labor day

it was like

Whitman's vision

on a global scale

as we scrambled to hold

Jürgen Habermas's glasses

when the sky changed

from bright blue

we moved everything

into the house

there are many good reasons

to wear a mask

teargas & toxic smoke

are just two

III.   the institution of the internet

the colonisation of cyberspace proceeds

online parks are the modern utopia

winding paths public spaces

                    colonial monuments

the views of the digital public

                    accord with ours

that monetisation has been

                    a universal good

IV.   thanks to new jersey

he filled the incubator / with concrete

& held a vigil / to mark the losses

V.   depressed people everywhere

suddenly we are all on zoom

faces speaking with micro audio delays

when the virus hit California

we self-consciously waved goodbye

our small world / suddenly smaller

VI.   screen freeze

we went to the doughnut store

for coffee

then flipped to Microsoft

it can't be too bad

getting lost in the US

limitless blue skies &

all those signs &

cheerful bumper stickers

easy to spell out

unmarked police cars

& armed vigilantes

to protect the vote

Covode 12: our little universe

4 john cooper clarke

I.   London demons

this was an unplanned voyage

despite the voices from mission control

whispering in our ears

after that ceremonial farewell

to soho

perhaps this was just an opportunity

to see us home safely

II.   at war

universities become laboratories

special advisers are history

despite the searchlight

some of the images have disappeared

but it's not hard to see

the fascist in front of you

10 years of collaboration

send the craft into a spin

but we still have the power

to observe the parallels

III.   the elegant mistakes

I can never disappear

I can never leave it alone

all poetry means restrictions

& the measures are already announced

if you're in this business

you can always work from home

it will be a treat

IV.   outside Minsk

it's wearing a balaclava, for example

or snatch patrols on the streets of Belarus

we have seen the films & read the books

we recognise the multiple uses of space

V.   the naked sky

the history of satellites is

a string of bright communications

invisible to the naked eye

the latest novelty spacecraft

recalibrates the heavens

the realm of the gods

with influence over us

is captured by machines

who tells us with images

what the future will be

VI.   to ease the pill

to ease the pill, as he puts it

he deploys laboratory staff

on the border question

in response to the local lockdown

we need never install a visor

the drugs drafted into the public realm

the reporters stand around the lighthouse

to find out the questions

that they never asked

VII.   stars are nice

there's a party vibe within the two camps

but the bars are closing

stars are nice

but they flood social media

while the satellite business

rewrites the night sky

the speed at which the virus orbits

is two weeks beyond intolerable

& London is like

some two or three days behind

we're incredibly excited

but will we be able to cope

with a ban on exclamations

VIII.   a new material engagement

we attend to the early stages

of human existence

a beguiling blend of manual

& verbal dexterity

he was one of the first home

with a velvety batch

of starlink underground news

before the potential

martini at teatime

he does his rock 'n' roll

swagger

on a collision course with time

IX.   the earth's atmosphere

with millions of dollars & trembling hands

maybe she isn't the most qualified

executive director, it's a knotty problem,

survivable possibly, with international

consequences, a tumble, perhaps,

that might compromise the space station,

capsule & cargo vehicles, a tumble that

takes us through space for ever

X.   celestial incarnations

traffic increased with time, satellites & space debris, blue skies
& contrails, then the rules of the road change, we lose the
megaconstellated way, with no time to collect data on other
frequencies

XI.   what pressures

while the great patriotic war is at hand, to hand NHS services,
monuments, street lights to private companies, years of partisan
testing, empty nightingale hospitals, & the prospect of a well-
funded army, set up to enforce English identity, pale corona-faces
breathing behind masks

XII.   downbeat

there have been no sustained protests

all this has become normal

heads turned back with a twist

after the build-up the hype & the fanfare

the emotional partings from wives & parents

the ritual beatings from security services

suffice to say, we are going to feel

black & blue later

XIII.   consequences

the searchlight falls on our little military vehicle, he hunches
forward for the interrogation in front of him, well, if Jack is
nervous about fighting ... this is not such a good situation, when
you look at it, 10 years of these memories of collaboration,
the war scenario could be a piece of schoolroom history,
or a rupture in the narratives of hundreds of museums, a
rapid depressurization, perhaps even a major catastrophe,
independence day is celebrated, but not on the day we were
liberated, we could send the craft back towards 1944, we could
raise a robotic arm, you could be left rotting in the old museum
complex, a defensive line built in the 1930s, back of the space
station, with consequences for the 21st century

Covode 13: et in arcadia ego

'when you want to screw everybody over all the time ... nobody wants
to buy anything from you'

I.   replicant capitalism

the style is part fluff, part

shoulderpads, part a portfolio

of high-street properties

billboards & skyscrapers

with a sound-track by Vangelis

grainy urban memories

well past their sell-by date

II.   the people's case

it's inconvenient to be tested

& impossible to give up work

it's out on the street, & the word

is added ad lib

(and not out of tenderness)

the struggle remains the same

III. politicians of our era

reflected neon & continuous rain

fugitive moments of futurist noir

all our contacts are shadows

the virus spread by a government

steeped in war-time nostalgia

for spivs & profiteers

the foot-soldiers self-isolate at home

confused about the enemy

IV. arcadia apartments

we are locked in our rooms

closer to the edge

quicker to the coming

into desires

brutal & terrifying

with an analyst

trying to make us share

the unnerving relevance

of fear

V.   more life

this rhetoric about choice

& freedom

there is a need to demand

what it means when someone

has turned

against being a functionary

of commodity fetishism

we do not gloss over

the product's contempt for us

those soft-porn

slow-motion advertisements

created by the magic

of sad magicians

we, too, rush to the box-office

VI.   on the run

understand this, we don't need

a Brechtian discourse of *Verfremdung*

the replicants are busy right now

they might even feel as we feel

that rich experience of living

that fairytale / that ends with a kiss

Covode 14: space milestones

I.   monolith

in this year of remote meetings

something that could be

produced by aliens

brought in by management

torn down by fundamentalists

II.   models on the beach

we have observed

the collapse

of an empire

amid hopes of escape

from the locked-down street

the infrastructural fig-leaf

of 'global britain'

for the slow walk down

to the job-centre

no mandate for unemployment

trade relations at a distance

don't compensate for the wrench

to companies markets specifications

now it's cash to chums

& better times

have to take their chances

III.   exchange rate

in this time of infection

with no real choices

but to follow the slow burn

& boost randomly back

Into the network

no match to set

the sky alight

no promise to sustain

artistic production

through public borrowing

to create a future

fit for 1950s Britain

IV.   about to crash

from primitive diptych

to multi-screen installations

visions of white

demonic make-up

along vistas of white

twisting roads

we suddenly come upon

the ghost of britain's reputation

in a no-deal Brexit

where no other country

ever infringes our sovereignty

V.   **walk / don't walk**

shot in the dark streets

with completely danceable rhythms

as if there were no

solo guitar interjections

the eye, likewise, more than viable

with nothing to do but jump

across the measurable gulfs of space

thinking about the elements

authority, the misuse of language

the lyrics, the videos that resonate

those little white lines with a litany

of swaggering pleasures with all

the appearance of torqueing of registers

& the sculptures, arms bent, to join him

on a violin tuned to the blues

they appear code red

his own back & arms run down

with zero inflammatory respite

déjà vu is a familiar response

to eke out so much with so few

contemporary constituent parts

white lines with plenty of space

it's hard not to salute / that particular idea

VI.   **the next corner**

midway through the clamour

breaks over us gagging

mouths for budget meals

as for the rest

it's only showing worse to come

VII.   robot ballet

15 miles east of the estuary

photography is strictly forbidden

there are private security guards

& the market is paranoid

it's impossible to forget this technology

it attacks the host

packets of noodles develop symptoms

before they can be put down

the future is flashed up on a screen

freezer-trucks outside the funeral home

body-bags where the citizens were

we're thankful we're on the latest chemicals

VIII.   treatment required

this looks like another bad day

I'm normally up in retail

for the arcadias we pastiche

need a range of suppliers

& recovery requires workers

to pick up your shopping

from a ventilator to a vaccine

there is no way this is likely

to give a subject access

to who really runs the shop

though projected wage cuts

send out unmistakable signals

IX.   gold standard

in an elliptical orbit

with prices & costs

protected by the heat-shield

then turned into a fire-ball

by inflationary measures that

trigger mass-strikes

& troops on the streets

the parachute will open

it will last a decade

X.   collapsed

with fingerprints on its gleaming surfaces, sullying its sound
finance, regardless of where it came from, a self-inflicted fiasco,
this new-wave framework, a light touch for hedge-funds, for
anything goes

XI.   space milestones

a kind of thrum sends our dreams

into over-drive – first a satellite

then our lunar base & a crewed space-station

third-country concerns about standards

are posted on instagram

forced to repeat the manoeuvre

space spills & tumbles

we fall between the one & the other

images of the beginnings of life

extra-terrestrials kick-start history

crowds on a burning plain

preprogrammed for migration

we return, broken down

our scientists hope the object

will help us to learn

the fate of humanity

Covode 15: something in the air

4 lynette yiadom-boakye

I.   **methodology**

a lot of random samples

fall into darkness

but a handful

of new variants

spread & go forwards

with renewed energy

II.   **modus operandi**

we experience / cognitive dissonance

the year keeps on doing / what it's doing

while a huge shadow hangs over us

a man can carry his documentation

as another anecdote for the archives

the man behind / is in paint-stained jeans

a third holds on to / the bigger picture

this one goes to the register of baptisms

this one is signed for at the door

this one carries the mark of his death

on his face

III.   first stop

then there are the painters

she admires

the immersive shiver

of bathers against waves

painting blackness

amidst the pandemonium

an eye, a cigarette behind an ear

hic incipit (meaning the plague)

political unrest on all sides

a language up against the wall

while those who still chronicle the city

walk towards a cinematic freeze-frame

IV.   preamble

yes, it is something

to write these poems

after all those deaths

that was something

he could not give

a final reconciliation

just metaphors & curses

for an infectious politics

& it gives us,

as it seems,

a heart, not ready

to rush into battle,

but this, he feels,

it can commit to

## V.	so this is the way

she had to go back to the futurists

the way Pound reprises Homer

& the plague comes to the viewer

while the family remains in the frame

a hairstyle a shoe a neckline

contemporary inexperience has made

this old aesthetic vocal

## VI.	debut

mouths mouth / in a baggy silence

it's never straightforward

though the result is /temporarily uplifting

it's hard to work

we measure with the eye

but the premise breaks

that much too comfortable conceit

VII.   lockdown

no bike rides round the city

now it's getting colder

instead, it's life

amid assorted images

all the advantages of the digital

we wanted a communal experience

it's what we are

programmed to do

to be with other bodies

just being

what they are

VIII.   the warning

tests are expected

there's every reason to believe

that they will work

we must be ready

despite the late notice

& the big business

of carrying out tests

privately

we try to remember the names

of those who have been killed

of those who have died

obliterated by this politics

he speaks of working photographs

as dramatic moments

the woman looks down, looks away

she doesn't speak, but she knows

we are an imagined community

not just wall-texts at the Tate.

Covode 16: a more perfect union

'aggressive boosterism is not naivety'

I.   game over

we thought there was a connection

between the height of hemlines

& the other end of the link

between the analysis / of vocal patterns

and the commentaries / on conspiracy theories

II.   star-dust

by the time you read this

the tribute concert will be over

an unholy alliance of Donald Trump

& that guy from down the road

the Thin White Duke

III.   **dress-rehearsal**

the virus might turn out

as skilful as influenza

at mutating

keeping the virus

in the community

could mean a regular carnival

of smashed windows

IV.   **critical care**

there are ventilators

vaccines

& we practice

social distancing

an elbow bump

provides a contact high

continuous party-mix music

of disco & 70's club culture

V.   the english variant

we all know what happens

in winter crises

it's a bit like a war

with the so-called commander

falling apart at the seams

we try to figure out

the latest version of the rules

taking it all / to another level

VI.   eton rifles

this is why we're in the mess we're in

the officer stands with his hands on the barrier

he grips the white shoulder & whispers

VII.   a significant scar

we expect machines / to manage the textual

& talk of how easily / the psyche is parsed

we try on personae, haircuts, poses

we create a character of cool creativity

we are targets for messages

forwarded by algorithms

Covode 17: after 100, 000 deaths

'how will we remember the plague that visited death upon us?'

I.   new community

we should be up for / face-to-face contact

we should provide / the sociologists

evidence of a new sociability

& some essential Joan Armatrading tracks

on old-school vinyl

in a dream of escape

from that familiar netherworld

to these pages / behind closed doors

where we're sitting

II.   repeat

the beeping, trying to silence

the beeping, after losing

another patient, I can't breathe

she says, & because of the beeping

she goes back, & tries to silence

the reasons for fear

III.   unknown duration

schoolwork goes on in isolation

she has what one might call

a disciplined brain

analytic skills

& old-school ideals

with digital access to the corpus

of English poetry

IV.   key principles

the infrastructure needed /to build on the flood plains

a website with a link / free at the point of use

& the name of the person / to manage

a privately-run service

there can still be debates / about 'levelling up'

& various measures called / 'supporting the economy'

you can speak to a cabinet minister

there's easy access / & guaranteed backbench support

you can cheer the return of former colleagues

& provide relief for colleagues' wives

V.   mailbox

a whole set of new procedures

& people I barely know

think it's ok to ask

for various favours

it turns out the brain

is on the receiving end

of all this harm

with cordoned-off sections

the cortex the striatum

disoriented after another email

from a former co-worker

while repeated task-switching

with a friend

raises levels of stress

VI.   commemoration

it's a philosophical project

like the mind-numbing numbers

of the dead

it's a grief suppressed

waiting for something to break

VII.   click on this

the film has been deferred

but denied your computer

you still try to manage

desensitization

& information reprocessing

making rhythmic eye-movements

(mail still sits in the box)

& much of our understanding

of action

& what we ask of others

(click on this)

the body's threat responses

such as negative concentration

in the face of really challenging

modes of communication

VIII.   gamestop

how will we remember

this anniversary

the funerals

via livestream

allow us to keep

our distance

without the consolation

of touch

in a year of

unremitting mourning

exchanges by

phone or letter

the vaccine frees me up

for contemplation

IX.   network I.

it's easy to succumb / silos of knowledge / called into collective
action / an armada of tiny killers /millions of copies /sweeps
through our cells / designed to latch on / to self-destruct / so the
long fight begins

X.   a localised outrage

one group in particular

can be encouraged

mobilised about the false

economy of bigotry

village style

but with all the amenities

of plastic ties

& military-grade weapons

that's what the project is

this time

XI. forgotten news

when this is over, remember

those signals from the top

(those distractions)

that characterise

the learning of lessons

the initial novelty

of emptied streets

of streets up-ended

let alone consolation

to make amends

for the pent-up sorrows

the horrors of long-running wars

of continuing famines

history suggests we may struggle

to find more than

dystopian markers

& maybe one last academic

freed from contagion guilt

will provide the narrative

discreet, private, abstract

Covode 18: out of this world

I.   new ballgame

there was no vegetation

no sign of life

only dust storms & winds

& millions of miles

from the nearest library

we play darts in the bar

we read through the system's history

we touch fingers to the screen

II.   deep impact

we have spent two years / in this thin atmosphere / capable of
sustaining investors / but no place for a dog / a 50kg robot rover
/ returning with samples / deep incisions in the crust / a slice of
real estate / with stunning overviews of Earth / & a potential for
development

III.   we remember

feeling worn out / in St Mark's Square

finding the Caffè Florian / closed

everything more difficult / than we had expected

IV.   moonshot

I'm obsessed with exploration

she says

the moon in her eyes

becomes another waste plot

V.   perfect seal

amid constant talk of

extra-terrestrials

& vaccines

we donned our / protective suits

that was the way we minimised

what it was really like

the truth becoming a blur

with all areas suddenly off limits

(we all knew someone who had died)

VI.   interlude

our conversations were clotted

with new terminology

our exchanges grew softer

as restrictions eased

then the second wave broke

with an end to the conversations

the walks across the fields

our lungs full of / cold city air

exhausted frustrated increasingly

emotional about / missed connections

we return to a baseline

knowledge of what closeness might be

VII.   a report on planetary protection

keep the anecdotes / for future times

we need to protect the survivors

we have been on assignment

to visit the most far-out sectors

water is a scarce resource

our constant restlessness

has damaged the surface rocks

VIII.   quantum uncertainty

it's a fact / that there is uncertainty

we wait patiently / & kill time

while our former colleagues / ignore our emails

if you're going to do Mars / just go for it

she handed in her notice

& started to feel human again

she wasn't sure she could sustain it

IX. among the masks

let's not forget our objectives

while we work more uncertainty

into the systems

there is therapy available

& counselling for the elderly

she had taken her leave / & returned to Earth

she had seriously considered / returning to the red planet

but declined the offer

it was a short-term apprenticeship

to death

X. disease prevention

so NASA sent us rocks / to learn from them

because laboratory samples on Earth

were contaminated

life brought back / into the biosphere

a microbial ripple effect

known as the Mars variant

XI.   the moon in your hand

for a long while

                                    the project felt precarious

investigations to mine gold

                                         & platinum

for evidence

                        of the Earth's present

now the oligarchs have arrived

& the celebrities are expected

                                 on site

there are no planning regulations

                                 or safety measures

we retreat into our cabins

                                 left to our own devices

XII.   simple time

lakes & mountains & glaciers

cross-country trips through ghost towns

                                    canyons

the best minds of my generation

                        in helmets goggles & facemasks

what knowledge of America

                            from brown bears & golden eagles

                            from soil samples

                            from wheels on icy Texas snow

XIII.   biosigns

the government has failed us

the voice announces / as the Board reconvenes

we have options / an escape plan

reorganising the city's demographics

occupying spaces vacated by the state

we are hiring for the project

it's another emerging market

a meteorite brought life

                           to small-town America

long before the dot.com crisis

our policy adviser

                           understands space advocacy

even if she's working

                           from California

Covode 19: out of the blue

4 paula rego

4 laura cumming

'arcadia is no more'

I.   am I blue?

we might know all the answers

but we still can't pay the bills

we mine for metals

inside dead computers

sift clear plastic

from organic waste

breathe the asbestos

from beached cargo ships

we've sold water & sky

to raise the cash

II.   tonic

familiar minor key variations

a standard blue ground

heartfelt subterranean blues

while meaningful yellows

unfold soft & sunlit

we are not in North London now

III.   road crew (blue period)

we had no word for homelessness

for foodbanks needed for survival

if blue is to signify the sea

& hospital gloves

this is the way to find

echoes in music

taking the lead

from the sound engineer

Picasso is driving

a forklift truck

he has tried retraining

during lockdown

while we eat

our way through our savings

IV.   arcadia is no more

we have witnessed the destruction

of 500 shops the hidden hand

in a latex glove

we have witnessed the dissolution

of an empire

the last renaissance painter

in robes of ultramarine

we have witnessed the transcendence

of online shopping

V. **portrait (2)**

we need this artifice   to recognise

different symptoms   in different interiors

the background of Manhattan   & fatigue

migraines   tingling in the arms & legs

these interlocking pieces   & all around them

problems multiplied   in low-toned blues

& the nervous system   ever-changing

blue finds a life   in palpitations

chest pains   metal fire-escapes

inflammation of moods   damage to the heart

VI.   the dominant

they experience dizziness

                     breathlessness

a stream of

          sub-atomic particles

run-offs from

          animal waste

& fertilisers

there's a price

          for intensive farming

algae blooms

          depletion of fish

                 & plants

VII.   disorientation

who orbits these colours / at a distance / an asteroid's surface / holds specks of soil / on a trajectory / grains of sand / millions of days

VIII.   biological diversity

we choose a device which allows

an ambitious sub-plot

for my more attentive comrades

a set of data points

digitised & lightly disguised

it's not neck-deep in water

it's not the head over the heels

it's not having no word

for foodbank

a blue water sound-track

of bubbles

loved-up in lockdown

this is the way / & finding it

is about as far as / every day

to make it visible

no previous convictions

but this is the way

to believing in Michael Gove

IX.   subdominant

as a result of human abstraction

there's a fine balance

in this colour-themed conclusion

we're dependent on blue

to send the message

& sometimes the vulnerabilities

of this colour

the difficulties of fixing

indigo for example

there's no time for coffee-breaks

& walks around the city

the excessive use of fertilisers

& antibiotics

the destruction of farmland

pollutants drained into rivers

we go home & talk

we try to make

the degraded soils

healthy again

our lifelong isolation

is another factor

X.   club nights

we are bedroom artists

elbow-deep in this / intimate music

a ghost-chain boy / out of his head

but not off his head

that vestige of discrimination

dates from a period / before facebook

he is finally in the picture

he feels love has come

pitch-shifted through the ease

knee-deep in the ghost-chain

knee-deep in the sale of product

mixing collaborating dismantling

this intimate music

a vestige of the night of first ages

this dream of the body

after lockdown comes to an end

XI.   assume form

he is positioned / in character

in his penthouse suite

for a documentary / about sexual consent

a dubstep producer turned / atmosphere writer

with a golden parachute / & his personal drone

he is made to tell us / exactly what happened

the solar wind strips off the cynicism

kicks off / a catalogue of damage

droughts & wildfires

traced to their point of origin

we can spot the difference

a kind of *quid pro quo*, for example

with a very specific global flavour

XII.   whisper rabbit

in this multi-tracked environment

we are comfortable with the ecstatic

for this textual happening

we waive our fears / & premonitions

for the chance of interconnectedness

not to dominate / with Disney strings

we are still paying for that melody

as we tiptoe through this moment

of public history

steroids will give us no protection

the skin of this living container

is thin & fragile

XIII.   catch

lest we forget

how mankind evolved

how they put us in a cage

how they dropped us

through the upper atmosphere

how they brought us back

the sample was not designed

to survive the return

but they will / create a document

this stream of proteins

this image of presence

still unsure / how to assume form

this capsule with its

payload of problems

XIV.   a distant anniversary

in 2018 the crew was invited

to descend safely / onto the test range

the data acquired / helped solve

several technical problems

our degraded script / reverberates

where soil has been lost

the blue ground, the unspoken

this thin layer of biofilm

this living skin

it's not too late

working 12-hour days

has raked the sparks

out of dying cinders

full circle back

to the ache of

wild swimming

the ease of

wild swimming

refracted synchronicities

in a game of chance

Robert Hampson

Afterword

My interest in the ode as a public voice poetry began a couple of years back with 'Ode: On Advance Booking', an attempt to up-date the classical form of the ode, inspired by the misreading of the heading on a document. These odes are structurally much freer - constellations of short sections for a multi-faceted moment. Many of them occupy particular places and inhabit a particular scenario including various enclosed spaces: submarines, bunkers, cruise ships, recording studios, space-stations.

2021

Biography: Robert Hampson

Robert Hampson was formerly Professor of Modern Literature in the Department of English at Royal Holloway, University of London. He is currently Professor Emeritus at Royal Holloway; Research Fellow at the Institute for English Studies, University of London; Visiting Professor at the University of Northumbria; and on the faculty of the New School of the Anthropocene.

He has been involved in the field of contemporary innovative poetry since the 1970s as editor, critic and practitioner. During the 1970s he co-edited the magazine *Alembic* with Peter Barry and Ken Edwards. He co-edited (with Peter Barry) the pioneering volume *New British poetries: The Scope of the Possible* (Manchester: Manchester University Press, 1993); and, more recently, has co-edited (with Will Montgomery) *Frank O'Hara Now* (Liverpool UP, 2010); (with Ken Edwards) *Clasp: late modernist poetry in London on the 1970s* (Shearsman 2016); and (with cris cheek) *The Allen Fisher Reader* (Shearsman 2020).

His own poetry has appeared in a range of magazines including Cid Corman's *Origin* and Alan Davies *100 Posters* in the 1970s. More recently, he has published poetry in *The Café Review, Long Poem Magazine, Junctionbox, Molly Bloom, Mercurius, parmenar, The Wolf, tentacular magazine*, and *Rewilding: an ecopoetic anthology* (2020). His early booklets included *degrees of addiction* (Share 1975); *How Nell Scored* (Poet and Peasant 1976); *a necessary displacement* (pushtika 1978); *a feast of friends* (Pig Press 1982); *A City at War* (Northern Lights 1985); *Nevsky Prospekt* (with David Miller) (hardPressed poetry 1988); *a human measure* (hardPressed poetry 1989); *unicorns: 7 studies in velocity* (pushtika 1989); *dingo* (with Gerlinde Roder-Bolton) (pushtika 1994); *seaport: interim edition* (pushtika 1995); *a new hampshire sampler* (with Gerlinde Roder-Bolton) (pushtika 1996); and the artist-book, *C for Security* (pushtika, 2001). *Assembled Fugitives: selected poems 1973-1998* was published by Stride (2001). His best-known work is *seaport* (Shearsman, 2008). More recent publications include *pentimento* (pushtika 2005); *an explanation of colours* (**Veer, 2010**); *the long view / wish you were here* (**artist-book with Leena Nammari**) (**2011**); *out of sight* (**Crater Press 2012**; *reworked disasters* (**Knives forks and spoons 2013**); and *Liverpool (hugs &) kisses* (**with Robert Sheppard**) (**ship of fools / pushtika 2015**).

He taught with Redell Olsen on the MA in Poetic Practice at Royal Holloway. For many years he ran the TALKS series that Bob Perelman set up in London, and has been co-running the Contemporary Innovative Poetry Research Seminar (which replaced it) ever since.

Biography: Joanna Levi

Joanna Levi studied music at Royal Holloway London University specialising in performance and gained a place for composition in the National Youth rchestra of Great Britain. However, she has always maintained a keen interest in composition, and hardly a day goes by without some form of practical composition for cello students. In this format she wrote a complete cello tutor in the format of cello duos. This project allowed a consuming interest in Bach's music to fuse with the inspirational poetry of the *Covodes* by Robert Hampson. Since composing the *Suite for Solo Cello*, Joanna Levi has written two more works for solo cello – one adhering to the Bachian theme, with a set of variations, the other nodding to a more contemporary dance format. Levi's next project is to take a Breugel painting as a starting point for a cello Concerto.

Comment from Levi on composing for *Covodes*:

"Robert Hampson had spent Lockdown charting the extraordinary experience in many diverse manifestations. The imagery and thoughts were too complex to depict in music, but the sense of numbness, of monotony and anxiety were possible to suggest. I took Bach's Suites for cello as a starting point, and distorted and pursued stretched tonality within dance metre to reflect the poetry. It follows the format of suite, with a Prelude, Allemande, Courante, Sarabande Bouree's and Gigue, but has an Epilogue, and one extra movement that has a reference to Bach's Fugue subject in F sharp minor which is very chromatic – again suggesting an unresolved and disturbed normality."

Joanna Levi, August, 2021

Biography: John Vernon Lord

The signed & numbered (20 copies) Art edition of *Covodes* by Robert Hampson features two tipped & signed art prints by John Vernon Lord in a 12" x 12" format, ISBN: 9781871671087.

John Vernon Lord (born 1939 in Derbyshire) is an author, illustrator and educator. He studied at Salford School of Art and at the Central School of Arts and Crafts in London. He has illustrated 40 books, his best-known works being *The Giant Jam Sandwich* (1972) and his award-winning edition of *The Nonsense Verse of Edward Lear* (1984), both published by Jonathan Cape and still in print. His children's books have been translated into many languages.

He has twice been the overall winner of the Victoria and Albert Museum Illustration Awards, with his *Aesop's Fables* in 1990 and for his illustrations in James Joyce's *Ulysses* in 2018, when he was awarded the Moira Gemmill Illustrator of the Year and the Best Illustrated Book prize.

Lord's illustrated edition of James Joyce's *Finnegan's Wake* was published by the Folio Society in 2014. Two monographs on his work have been published – *Drawing Upon Drawing* (2007) and *Drawn to Drawing* (2014). Lord has illustrated the Folio Society's *Myths and Legends of the British Isles*, *Icelandic Sagas*, and *Epics of the Middle Ages*. In addition he has illustrated several classics of children's literature, including Lewis Carroll's *Alice's Adventures in Wonderland* (2009), *Through the Looking Glass* (2011), and *The Hunting of the Snark* (2006), published by Artists' Choice Editions. Among the 40 books he has illustrated, 15 of them are children's books including 4 of his own stories.

Lord has lectured on the art of illustration in the UK and internationally for the past 60 years. He was chair of the Graphic Design Board of the Council for Academic Awards during the 1980s, and he is Professor Emeritus at the University of Brighton, having been Professor of Illustration there from 1986 where he taught from 1961 to 1999. An Honorary DLitt was conferred upon him by the University of Brighton in 2000.

Biography: Patricia Hope Scanlan

Patricia Hope Scanlan (born 1958) in Ireland and has worked in England since 1983, Winner of the Guinness Prize for Poetry from Seamus Heaney in 1982 (Maynooth); returning to Ireland in 1988 to organize an all-Ireland *Poets Convention* in Cork, launching the publishing house Ink Sculptors at this time. Back in England, Scanlan was Literary Editor of *Casablanca* Magazine, founder & co-editor of *Lovely Jobly*: International Arts Magazine (1989-1991) run by artists, organizing exhibitions and arts events in London. She founded a magazine *SuperReal* charting surreal influences in English literature & the arts, & curated a British Surrealism Exhibition (East West Gallery, London). Her collections of poems include *Selected Poems* published (Tuba Press, 1993), *Yell ow, Three Dimensional Sin* (Ink Sculptors, 1988) working with what she described as 'Power Texts'; *A Picture of Water* (1991); *Hasting, Hastings* (Our Wonderful Culture, 1990); the collections *The Trees are Moving to China and Taking the Sun as a Leaf* (2008), *I Dreamt of Daniel Boone* (1996), and *Fassbinder's Still Lives*, 2000 (all published by Joe DiMaggio Press) and *Reeling in Slow Motion* (Pressed Wafer, Boston, 2002); her most recent collection *Nature is the Hardest Thing of All or Not Made in China* (2020) published by Tuba Press. Since the late-90s, Scanlan has worked making Performance Art works, and has relaunched Artery Editions to collaborate with artists & writers. *Earthworks*, an occasional magazine championing work celebrating our planet, 2021, appearing under the Artery Editions umbrella.

Biography: Cameron Macgregor

Cameron Macgregor (born 2000 in Edinburgh) is a freelance creative, writer, poet, and professional tutor based in Bristol, generally creating work exploring experimental theatre. Macgregor runs a Covid-bourne digital theatre company, *Theatre-19*, performing at Edinburgh Fringe Festival 2021. Macgregor volunteers for charities across Bristol and works on administration and sound design for Artery Editions.

Biography: Clare Davey

Clare Davey (born Scotland, 1967), is a freelance designer and digital skills tutor based in Brighton & Hove. Clare has worked in the design industry for over 25 years working for a major London local authority, the Museum of London and the BBC where she was promoted to Design Manager. Clare trained at the Glasgow School of Art, graduating with a first class degree in graphic design. She then went on to continue her education at the Royal College of Art, London completing an MA in graphic design.